Keto Chaffle Cookbook

50 wonderful recipes to have fun in the kitchen

Catherine Willis

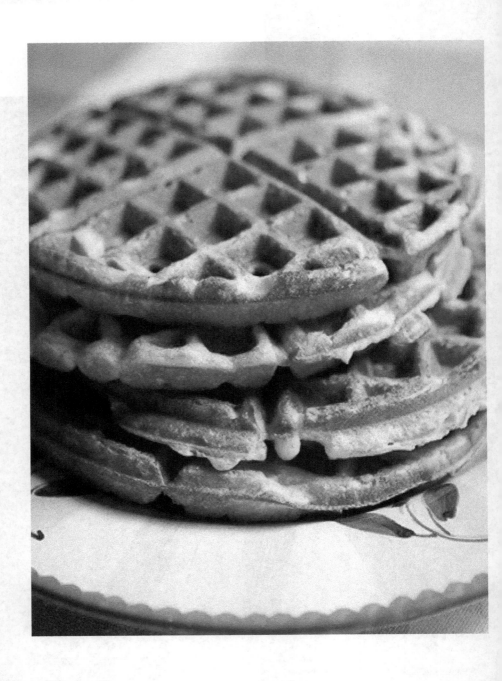

sources. Please consult a licensed professional before attempting any techniques outlined in this book.

By reading this document, the reader agrees that under no circumstances is the author responsible for any losses, direct or indirect, which are incurred as a result of the use of information contained within this document, including, but not limited to, — errors, omissions, or inaccuracies.

Table of Contents

Chicken Bites with Chaffles

Preparation time : 10 minutes

Cooking Time : 10 minutes

Servings : 2

INGREDIENTS:

1 chicken breasts cut into 2 x2 inch chunks

1 egg, whisked

1/4 cup almond flour

2 tbsps. onion powder

2 tbsps. garlic powder

1 tsp. dried oregano

1 tsp. paprika powder

1 tsp. salt

1/2 tsp. black pepper

2 tbsps. avocado oil

DIRECTIONS:

1. Together, apply all of the dry ingredients to a large bowl. Mix thoroughly.
2. Place them in a separate bowl with the eggs.
3. Dip each piece of chicken into the egg, then into the dry ingredients.
4. Heat oil in a 10-inch skillet, add oil.

5. Once avocado oil is hot, place the coated chicken nuggets onto a skillet and cook for 6-8 minutes until golden brown.

6. Serve with chaffles and raspberries.

NUTRITION : Total Calories: 401kcal Fats: 219g Protein: 32.35g Fiber: 3g

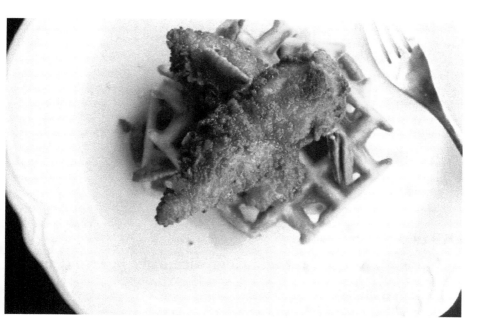

Crunchy Fish and Chaffle Bites

Servings :4

Cooking Time : 15 Minutes

INGREDIENTS :

  1 lb. cod fillets, sliced into 4 slice

  1 tsp. sea salt

  1 tsp. garlic powder

  1 egg, whisked

  1 cup almond flour

  2 tbsp. avocado oil

  CHAFFLE Ingredients:

  2 eggs

  1/2 cup cheddar cheese

  2 tbsps. almond flour

  ½ tsp. Italian seasoning

DIRECTIONS:

1. Mix together chaffle ingredients in a bowl and make 4 square

2. Put the chaffles in a preheated chaffle maker.

3. Mix together the salt, pepper, and garlic powder in a mixing bowl. Toss the cod cubes in this mixture and let sit for 10 minutes.

4. Then dip each cod slice into the egg mixture and then into the almond flour.

5. Heat oil in skillet and fish cubes for about 2-3 minutes, until cooked and browned
6. Serve on chaffles and enjoy!

NUTRITION : Protein: 121kcal Fat: 189kcal Carbohydrates: 11kcal

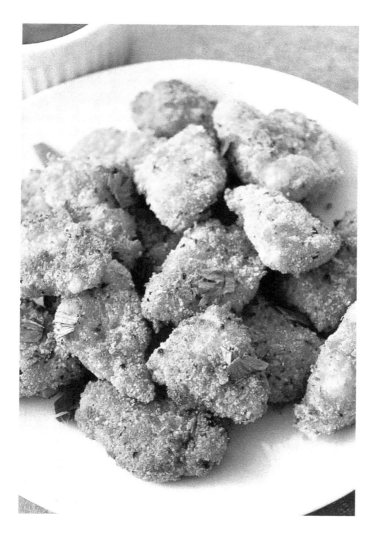

Grill Pork Chaffle Sandwich

Preparation time : 10 minutes

Servings :2

Cooking Time : 15 Minutes

INGREDIENTS :

1/2 cup mozzarella, shredded

1 egg

I pinch garlic powder

PORK PATTY

1/2 cup pork, minutes

1 tbsp. green onion, diced

1/2 tsp Italian seasoning

Lettuce leaves

DIRECTIONS :

1. Preheat the square waffle maker and grease with
2. Mix together egg, cheese and garlic powder in a small mixing bowl.
3. Pour batter in a preheated waffle maker and cover.
4. Make 2 chaffles from this batter.
5. Cook chaffles for about 2-3 minutes Utes until cooked through.
6. Meanwhile, mix together pork patty ingredients in a bowl and make 1 large patty.

7. Grill pork patty in a preheated grill for about 3-4 minutes Utes per side until cooked through.

8. Arrange pork patty between two chaffles with lettuce leaves. Cut the sandwich to make a triangular sandwich.

NUTRITION : Protein: 85 kcal Fat: 86 kcal Carbohydrates: 7 kcal

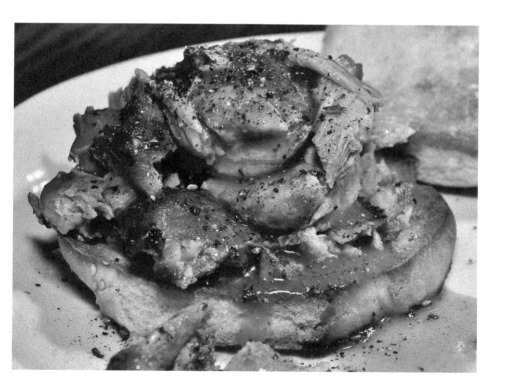

Chaffe & Chicken Lunch Plate

Preparation time : 10 minutes

Servings: 2

Cooking Time : 15 Minutes

INGREDIENTS:

1 large egg

1/2 cup jack cheese, shredded

1 pinch salt

For Serving

1 chicken leg

Salt

Pepper

1 tsp. garlic, minutes

1 egg

1 tsp avocado oil

DIRECTIONS:

1. Heat your square waffle maker and grease with cooking spray.
2. Pour Chaffle batter into the skillet and cook for about 3 minutes.
3. Put a pan over medium heat and heat the oil.
4. Once the oil is hot, add chicken thigh and garlic then, cook for about 5 minutes. Flip and cook for another 3-4 minutes.

5. Season with salt and pepper and mix well.
6. Transfer cooked thigh to plate.
7. Fry the egg in the same pan for about 1-2 minutes.
8. Once chaffles are cooked, serve with fried egg and chicken thigh.
9. Enjoy!

NUTRITION : Protein: 31% Fat: 66% Carbohydrates: 2%

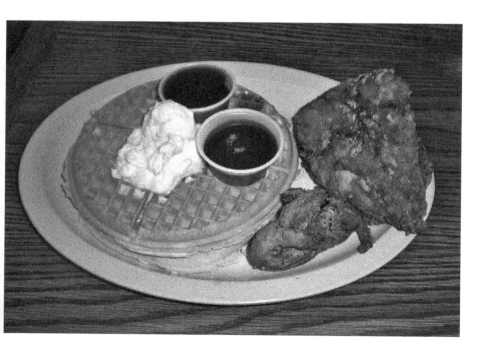

Chaffle Egg Sandwich

Preparation time : 10 minutes

Cooking Time : 10 Minutes

Servings :2

INGREDIENTS:

2 minutes keto chaffle

2 slice cheddar cheese

1 egg simple omelet

DIRECTIONS :

1. Prepare your oven at 400°F.
2. Arrange egg omelet and cheese slice between chaffles.
3. Cook for about 4-5 minutes in the preheated oven until the cheese has melted.
4. Once the cheese is melted, remove from the oven.
5. Serve and enjoy!

NUTRITION : Protein: 144kcal Fat: 337kcal Carbohydrates: 14kcal

..

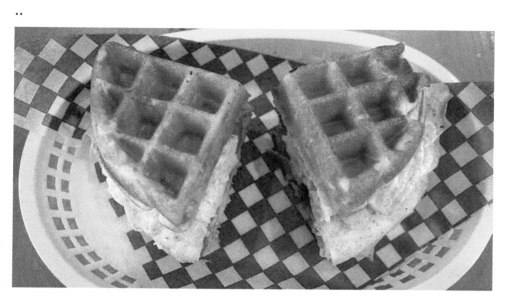

Chaffle Minutes Sandwich

Preparation time : 10 minutes

Cooking Time: 10 Minutes

Servings : 2

INGREDIENTS:

1 large egg

1/8 cup almond flour

1/2 tsp. garlic powder

3/4 tsp. baking powder

1/2 cup shredded cheese

SANDWICH FILLING

2 slices deli ham

2 slices tomatoes

1 slice cheddar cheese

DIRECTIONS:

1. Grease your square waffle maker and preheat it on medium heat.
2. Mix together chaffle ingredients in a mixing bowl until well combined.
3. Pour batter into a square waffle and make two chaffles.
4. Once chaffles are cooked, remove from the maker.
5. For a sandwich, arrange deli ham, tomato slice and cheddar cheese between two chaffles.

6. Cut sandwich from the center.

7. Serve and enjoy!

NUTRITION : Protein: 70kcal Fat: 159kcal Carbohydrates: 10kcal

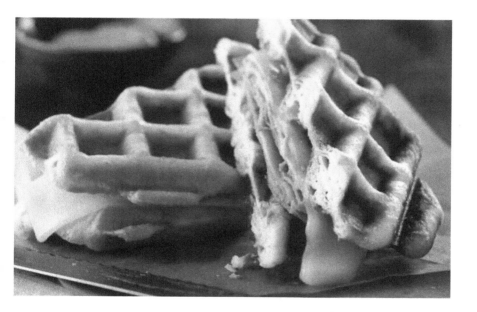

Chaffle Cheese Sandwich

Preparation time : 10 minutes

Servings: 1

Cooking Time : 10 Minutes

INGREDIENTS:

2 square keto chaffle

2 slice cheddar cheese

2 lettuce leaves

DIRECTIONS:

1. Prepare your oven at 400°F.
2. Arrange lettuce leaves and cheese slices between chaffles.
3. Cook for about 4-5 minutes in the preheated oven until the cheese has melted.
4. Once the cheese is melted, remove from the oven.
5. Serve and enjoy!

NUTRITION : Protein: 28% Fat: 69% Carbohydrates: 3 %

Chicken Zinger Chaffle

Preparation time : 10 minutes

Servings :2

Cooking Time : 15 Minutes

INGREDIENTS:

1 chicken breast, cut into 2 pieces

1/2 cup coconut flour

1/4 cup finely grated Parmesan

1 tsp. paprika

1/2 tsp. garlic powder

1/2 tsp. onion powder

1 tsp. salt & pepper

1 egg beaten

Avocado oil for frying

Lettuce leaves

BBQ sauce

Chaffle Ingredients:

4 oz. cheese

2 whole eggs

2 oz. almond flour

1/4 cup almond flour

1 tsp baking powder

DIRECTIONS:

1. Mix together chaffle ingredients in a bowl.

2. Pour the chaffle batter in a preheated greased square waffle maker.
3. Cook chaffles for about 2-minutes utes until cooked through.
4. Make square chaffles from this batter.
5. Meanwhile mix together coconut flour, parmesan, paprika, garlic powder, onion powder salt and pepper in a bowl.
6. Dip chicken first in coconut flour mixture then in beaten egg.
7. Heat avocado oil in a skillet and cook chicken from both sides. until lightly brown and cooked
8. Set chicken zinger between two chaffles with lettuce and BBQ sauce.
9. Enjoy!

NUTRITION : Protein: 219kcal Fat: 435kcal Carbohydrates: 66kcal

Double Chicken Chaffles

Preparation time : 10 minutes

Servings :2

Cooking Time: 5 Minutes

INGREDIENTS:

1/2 cup boiled shredded chicken

1/4 cup cheddar cheese

1/8 cup parmesan cheese

1 egg

1 tsp. Italian seasoning

1/8 tsp. garlic powder

1 tsp. cream cheese

DIRECTIONS :

1. Preheat the Belgian waffle maker.
2. Mix together in chaffle ingredients in a bowl and mix together.
3. Sprinkle 1 tbsp. of cheese in a waffle maker and pour in chaffle batter.
4. Pour 1 tbsp. of cheese over batter and cover.
5. Cook chaffles for about 4 to minutes Utes.
6. Serve with a chicken zinger and enjoy the double chicken flavor.

NUTRITION : Protein: 60 kcal Fat: 129kcal Carbohydrates: 9kcal

Chaffles With Topping

Preparation time : 10 minutes

Cooking Time: 10 Minutes

INGREDIENTS:

1 large egg

1 tbsp. almond flour

1 tbsp. full-fat Greek yogurt

1/8 tsp baking powder

1/4 cup shredded Swiss cheese

TOPPING

4oz. grill prawns

4 oz. steamed cauliflower mash

1/2 zucchini sliced

3 lettuce leaves

1 tomato, sliced

1 tbsp. flax seeds

DIRECTIONS:

1. Make 3 chaffles with the given chaffles ingredients.
2. For serving, arrange lettuce leaves on each chaffle.
3. Top with zucchini slice, grill prawns, cauliflower mash and a tomato slice.
4. Drizzle flax seeds on top.
5. Serve and enjoy!

NUTRITION : Protein: 71kcal Fat: 75kcal Carbohydrates: 12kcal

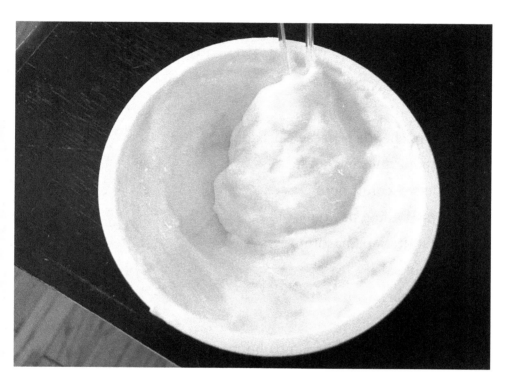

Chaffle With Cheese & Bacon

Preparation time : 10 minutes

Servings :2

Cooking Time : 15 Minutes

INGREDIENTS:

1 egg

1/2 cup cheddar cheese, shredded

1 tbsp. parmesan cheese

3/4 tsp coconut flour

1/4 tsp baking powder

1/8 tsp Italian Seasoning

pinch of salt

1/4 tsp garlic powder

FOR TOPPING

1 bacon sliced, cooked and chopped

1/2 cup mozzarella cheese, shredded

1/4 tsp parsley, chopped

DIRECTIONS:

1. Preheat the oven to 400 degrees.
2. Switch on your minutes waffle maker and grease with cooking spray.
3. Mix together chaffle ingredients in a mixing bowl until combined.

4. Spoon half of the batter in the center of the waffle maker and cover. Cook chaffles for about 3-minutes until cooked.
5. Carefully remove chaffles from the maker.
6. Arrange chaffles in a greased baking tray.
7. Top with mozzarella cheese, chopped bacon and parsley.
8. And bake in the oven for 4 -5 minutes.
9. Once the cheese is melted, remove from the oven.
10. Serve and enjoy!

NUTRITION : Protein: 28% Fat: 69% Carbohydrates: 3%

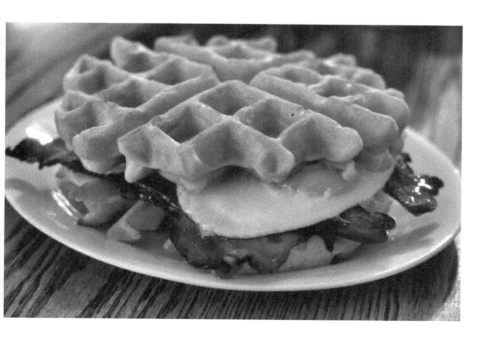

Grill Beefsteak and Chaffle

Preparation time : 10 minutes

Servings : 1

Cooking Time: 10 Minutes

INGREDIENTS:

  1 beefsteak rib eye

  1 tsp salt

  1 tsp pepper

  1 tbsp. lime juice

  1 tsp garlic

DIRECTIONS:

1. Prepare your grill for direct heat.
2. Mix together all spices and rub over beefsteak evenly.
3. Set the beef over medium heat on the grill rack..
4. Cover and cook steak for about6 to 8 minutes Utes. Flip and cook for another 5 minutes until cooked.
5. Serve with a simple keto chaffle and enjoy!

NUTRITION : Protein: 274kcal Fat: 243kcal Carbohydrates: 22kcal

Cauliflower Chaffles And Tomatoes

Preparation time : 10 minutes

Servings :2

Cooking Time: 15 Minutes

INGREDIENTS:

1/2 cup cauliflower

1/4 tsp. garlic powder

1/4 tsp. black pepper

1/4 tsp. Salt

1/2 cup shredded cheddar cheese

1 egg

FOR TOPPING

1 lettuce leaf

1 tomato sliced

4 oz. cauliflower steamed, mashed

1 tsp sesame seeds

DIRECTIONS:

1. Add all chaffle ingredients into a blender and mix well.

2. Sprinkle 1/8 shredded cheese on the waffle maker and pour cauliflower mixture in a preheated waffle maker and sprinkle the rest of the cheese over it.

3. Cook chaffles for about 4-5 minutes until cooked

4. For serving, lay lettuce leaves over the chaffle top with steamed cauliflower and tomato.

5. Drizzle sesame seeds on top.

NUTRITION : Protein: 49kcal Fat: 128kcal Carbohydrates: 21kcal

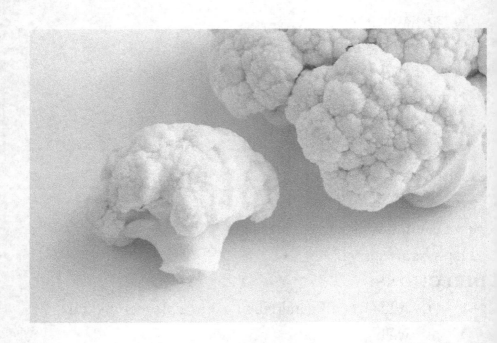

Breakfast chaffle sandwich

Preparation Time : 5 minutes

Cooking Time: 15 minutes

Servings : 1

INGREDIENTS:

1 egg

1/2 cup monterey jack cheese

1 tbsp almond flour

2 tbsp butter

DIRECTIONS:

1. Preheat the waffle maker for 5 minutes.
2. Combine monterey jack cheese, almond flour, and the egg in a bowl.
3. Take 1/2 of the batter and pour it into the preheated waffle maker. Allow to cook for 3-4 minutes.
4. Repeat the previous step for the remaining batter.
5. Melt butter on a small pan. Just like you would with French toast, add the chaffles and let each side cook for 2 minutes. To make them crispier, press down on the chaffles while they cook.
6. Remove the chaffles from the pan. Allow to cool.

NUTRITION :

Calories: 514Cal

Total Fat: 47g

Cholesterol: 0mg

Sodium: 0mg

Total Carbs: 0g

Sugar: 0g

Protein: 21g

Peanut butter and jelly chaffles

Preparation Time : 5 minutes

Cooking Time: 15 minutes

Servings: 1

INGREDIENTS:

1 egg

2 slices cheese, thinly sliced

1 tsp natural peanut butter

1 tsp sugar-free raspberry

Cooking spray

DIRECTIONS:

1. Crack and whisk the egg in a small bowl
2. Preheat and spray the waffle maker.
3. Once it is heated up, place a slice of cheese on the waffle maker and wait for it to melt.
4. Once melted, pour the egg mixture onto the melted cheese.
5. Once the egg starts cooking, carefully place another slice of cheese on the waffle maker.
6. Cover. Cook for 3-4 minutes.
7. Take out the chaffles and place on a plate.
8. Top the chaffles with whipped cream.

9. Drizzle some natural peanut butter and raspberry on top.

NUTRITION :

Calories: 337Cal

Total Fat: 27g

Saturated Fat: 0g

Total Carbs: 3g

Protein: 21g

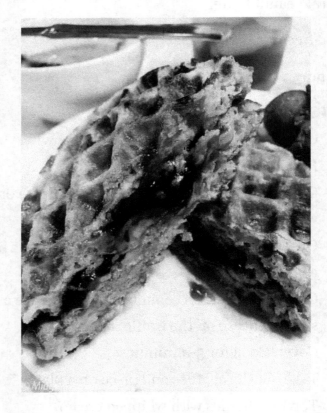

Halloumi cheese chaffles

Preparation Time : 5 minutes

Cooking Time: 10 minutes

Servings : 1

INGREDIENTS:

3 oz halloumi cheese

2 tbsp pasta sauce

DIRECTIONS:

1. Make half-inch thick slices of halloumi cheese.
2. With the waffle maker still turned off, place the cheese slices on it.
3. Turn on the waffle maker and let the cheese cook for 3-6 minutes.
4. Remove from the waffle maker and let it cool.
5. Add low-carb pasta or marinara sauce.

NUTRITION :

Calories: 333Cal

Total Fat: 26g

Saturated Fat: 0g

Cholesterol: 0mg

Total Carbs: 2g

Protein: 22g

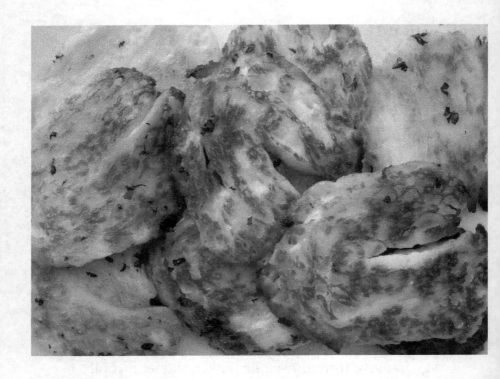

Breakfast Chaffle

Prep time: 5 min.

Cook time : 5 min.

Servings : 2

INGREDIENTS :

2 eggs

½ cup shredded mozzarella cheese

FOR THE TOPPINGS:

2 ham slices

1 fried egg

DIRECTIONS:

1. Mix eggs and cheese in a small bowl.

2. Turn on the waffle maker to heat and oil it with cooking spray. Onto the waffle maker, add half of the batter.

3. Cook for 2-4 minutes, remove, and repeat with remaining batter. Place egg and ham between two chaffles to make a sandwich.

NUTRITION :

Carbs: 1g, Fat: 8g Protein: 9g Calories: 115kcal

Carnivore chaffle

Preparation Time : 5 minutes

Cooking Time: 10 minutes

Servings: 1

INGREDIENTS:

1 egg

1/3 cup mozzarella cheese

1/2 cup pork rinds

Salt

DIRECTIONS:

1. Preheat the waffle maker.
2. In a small mixing bowl, mix a pinch of salt with the cheese, egg, and pork rinds.
3. Pour the mixture onto the preheated waffle maker. Cover and wait for 3-5 minutes while it cooks. You'll know it's cooked once it already has a golden-brown color.
4. Carefully remove it from the waffle maker and **Servings** .

NUTRITION :

Calories: 274Cal

Total Fat: 20g

Saturated Fat: 0g

Cholesterol: 0mg

Total Carbs: 1g

Protein: 23g

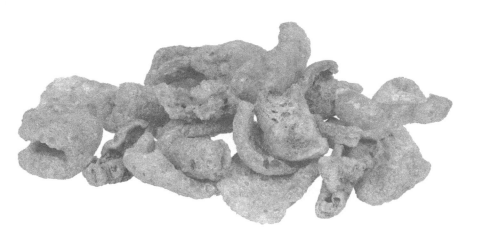

Cauliflower chaffle

Preparation time : 5 minutes

Cooking time: 5 minutes

Servings : 1

INGREDIENTS:

1/2 cup of rice cauliflower

1/4 shredded cheddar

1 large egg from which half of the yolk has been removed

1 tbsp fine almond flour

Salt and pepper

Sprinkle extra cheese on the bottom.

DIRECTIONS:

1. spread the mix on a waffle iron and add more cheese.
2. Cook for 8 minutes.

NUTRITION :

Calories: 200Cal

Total Fat: 16g

Saturated Fat: 0g

Cholesterol: 0mg

Total Carbs: 2g

Fiber: 2g

Protein: 11g

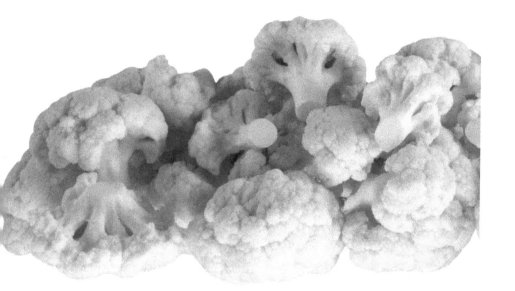

Hot Dog Chaffles

Preparation Time : 15 minutes

Cooking Time: 14 minutes

Servings: 2

INGREDIENTS:

1 egg, beaten

1 cup finely grated cheddar cheese

2 hot dog sausages, cooked

Mustard dressing for topping

8 pickle slices

DIRECTIONS :

1. Preheat the waffle iron.
2. In a medium bowl, mix the egg and cheddar cheese.
3. Open the iron and add half of the mixture. Close and cook until crispy, 7 minutes.
4. Transfer the chaffle to a plate and make a second chaffle in the same manner.
5. To serve, top each chaffle with a sausage, swirl the mustard dressing on top, and then divide the pickle slices on top.

NUTRITION :

Calories: 231Cal

Total Fat: 18.29g

Saturated Fat: 0g

Cholesterol: 0mg

Total Carbs: 2.8g

Protein: 13.39g

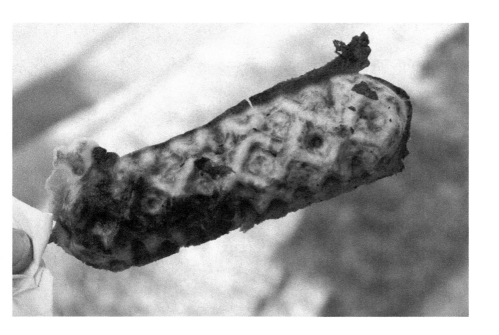

Omelette

Preparation Time : 8 minutes

Cooking Time : 17 minutes

Servings : 2

INGREDIENTS :

7 ounces of spinach (frozen)

6 large eggs

2 tablespoons of milk

2 teaspoons oil

A single tablespoon of herbs

¼ cup grated sharp cheddar

1/4 cup grated parmesan cheese

¼ cup crumbled, mild feta cheese

1 handful kale, chopped

½ cup ricotta cheese

Pepper for taste

DIRECTIONS :

1. Ensure there is no liquid in your spinach.
2. Chop the spinach finely then do the same with the kale.

3. Add the parmesan cheese along with cheddar, eggs, and milk and mix well.
4. Mix the herbs, feta, and ricotta in a separate bowl and then season with pepper.
5. Place the bowl to the side.
6. Heat a single teaspoon of olive oil in a pan that is non-stick.
7. Pour in half of the egg mix you made.
8. On medium-high heat fry until just set.
9. Add half of the ricotta mix on top before folding the omelette over.
10. Place a lid over the pan and then cook for another minute so that your filling is warmed.
11. Repeat for the second omelette.

NUTRITION :

Calories: 522Cal

Total Fat: 34.7g

Saturated Fat: 0g

Cholesterol: 0mg

Total Carbs: 10.3g

Fiber: 2.4g

Protein: 44 g

Pandan Asian Chaffles

Preparation Time : 3 minutes

Cooking Time : 8 minutes

Servings : 2

INGREDIENTS :

½ cup cheddar cheese, finely shredded

1 egg

3 drops of pandan extract

1 tbsp almond flour

1/3 tsp garlic powder

DIRECTIONS :

1. Warm up your mini waffle maker.
2. Mix the egg, almond flour, garlic powder with cheese in a small bowl.
3. Add pandan extract to the cheese mixture and mix well.
4. For a crispy crust, add a teaspoon of shredded cheese to the waffle maker and cook for 30 seconds.
5. Pour and cook the mixture in the waffle maker for 5 minutes.
6. Repeat with remaining batter.
7. Serve with fried chicken wings with bbq sauce.

NUTRITION :

Calories: 170Cal

Total Fat: 13g

Saturated Fat: 0g

Cholesterol: 0mg

Total Carbs: 2g

Protein: 11g

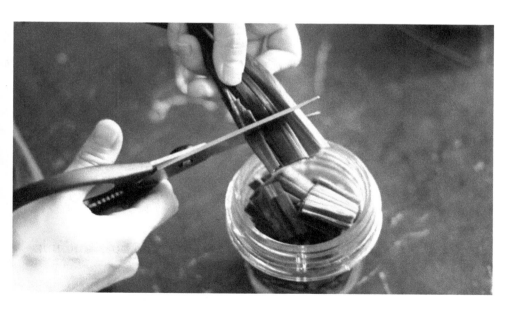

Ham and Jalapenos Chaffle

Preparation Time : 5 minutes

Cooking Time : 9 minutes

Servings : 3

INGREDIENTS :

2 lbs cheddar cheese, finely grated

2 large eggs

½ jalapeno pepper, finely grated

2 ounces ham steak

1 medium scallion

2 tsp coconut flour

DIRECTIONS:

1. Shred the cheddar cheese using a fine grater.
2. Deseed a jalapeno and grate using the same grater.
3. Finely chop the scallion and ham.
4. Pour all the ingredients in a medium bowl and mix well.
5. Spray your waffle iron with cooking spray and heat for 3 minutes.
6. Pour 1/4 of the batter mixture into the waffle iron.
7. Cook for 3 minutes, until crispy around the edges.

8. Remove the waffles from the heat and repeat until all the batter is finished.

9. Once done, allow them to cool and enjoy.

NUTRITION :

Calories: 120Cal

Total Fat: 10g

Saturated Fat: 0g

Cholesterol: 0mg

Total Carbs: 2g

Protein: 12g

Hot Ham Chaffles

Preparation Time : 5 minutes

Cooking Time : 4 minutes

Servings : 4

INGREDIENTS :

½ cup mozzarella cheese, shredded

1 egg

¼ cup ham, chopped

¼ tsp salt

2 tbsp mayonnaise

1 tsp Dijon mustard

DIRECTIONS :

1. Preheat your waffle iron.
2. In the meantime, add the egg in a small mixing bowl and whisk.
3. Mix-in the ham, cheese, and salt.
4. Scoop half the mixture using a spoon and pour into the hot waffle iron.
5. Close and cook for 4 minutes.
6. Remove the waffle and place on a large plate. Repeat the process with the remaining batter.

7. In another bowl, add the mustard and mayo. Mix together until smooth.
8. Slice the waffles in quarters and use the mayo mixture as the dip.

NUTRITION :

Calories: 110Cal

Total Fat: 12g

Saturated Fat: 0g

Cholesterol: 0mg

Total Carbs: 6g

Protein: 12g

Bacon & Egg Chaffles

Preparation Time : 5 minutes

Cooking Time : 10 minutes

Servings : 2

INGREDIENTS :

2 eggs

4 tsp collagen peptides, grass-fed

2 tbsp pork panko

3 slices crispy bacon

DIRECTIONS:

1. Warm up your mini waffle maker.
2. Combine the eggs, pork panko, and collagen peptides. Mix well. Divide the batter in two small bowls.
3. Once done, evenly distribute ½ of the crispy chopped bacon on the waffle maker.
4. Pour one bowl of the batter over the bacon. Cook for 5 minutes and immediately repeat this step for the second chaffle.
5. Plate your cooked chaffles and sprinkle with extra Panko for an added crunch.

NUTRITION :

Calories: 266Cal

Total Fat: 17g

Saturated Fat: 0g

Cholesterol: 0mg

Total Carbs: 11.2g

Protein: 27g

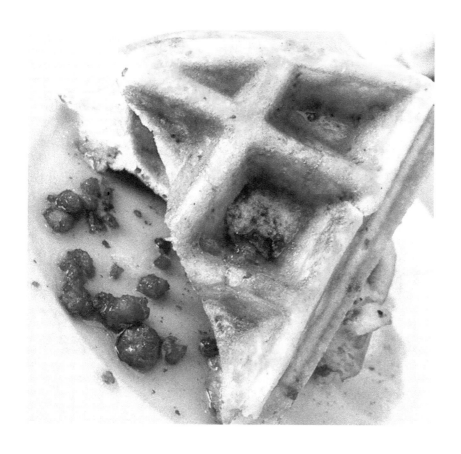

Cheese-free Breakfast Chaffle

Preparation Time : 4 minutes

Cooking Time : 12 minutes

Servings : 1

INGREDIENTS :

1 egg

½ cup almond milk ricotta, finely shredded.

1 tbsp almond flour

2 tbsp butter

DIRECTIONS :

1. Mix the egg, almond flour and ricotta in a small bowl.
2. Separate the chaffle batter into two and cook each for 4 minutes.
3. Pour on top of the chaffles, the melted butter.
4. Put them back in the pan and cook on each side for 2 minutes.
5. Remove from the pan and allow them sit for 2 minutes.
6. Enjoy while still crispy.

NUTRITION :

Calories: 530Cal

Total Fat: 50g

Saturated Fat: 0g

Cholesterol: 0mg

Total Carbs: 3g

Protein: 23g

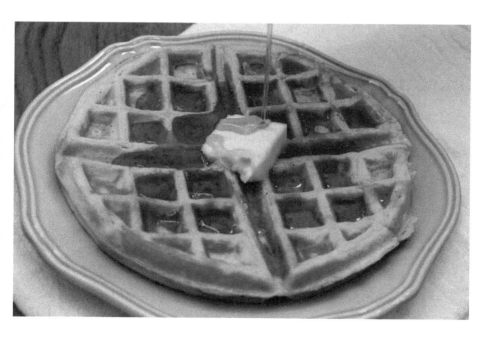

Bacon Chaffle Omelettes

Preparation Time : 5 minutes

Cooking Time : 10 minutes

Servings : 2

INGREDIENTS :

2 slices bacon, raw

1 egg

1 tsp maple extract, optional

1 tsp all spices

DIRECTIONS :

1. Put the bacon slices in a blender and turn it on.
2. Once ground up, add in the egg and all spices. Go on blending until liquefied.
3. Heat your waffle maker on the highest setting and spray with non-stick cooking spray.
4. Introduce half the omelette into the waffle maker and cook for 5 minutes max.
5. Remove the crispy omelette and repeat the same steps with rest batter.
6. Enjoy the warmth.

NUTRITION :

Calories: 59Cal

Total Fat: 4.4g

Saturated Fat: 0g

Total Carbs: 1g

Protein: 5g

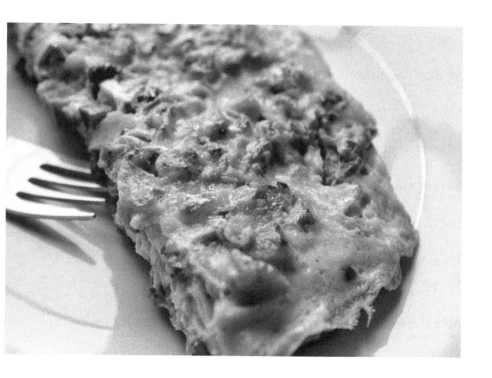

Avocado Chaffle Toast

Preparation Time : 4 minutes

Cooking Time : 8 minutes

Servings : 2

INGREDIENTS :

½ avocado

1 egg

½ cup cheddar cheese, finely shredded

1 tbsp almond flour

1 tsp lemon juice, fresh

Salt, ground pepper to taste

Parmesan cheese, finely shredded for garnishing

DIRECTIONS:

Warm up your mini waffle maker.

Mix the egg, almond flour with cheese in a small bowl.

For a crispy crust, add a teaspoon of shredded cheese to the waffle maker and cook for 30 seconds.

To the waffle maker, add the mixture and cook for 5 minutes.

Repeat with remaining batter.

Mash avocado with a fork until well combined and add lemon juice, salt, pepper

Top each chaffle with avocado mixture. Sprinkle with parmesan and enjoy!

NUTRITION :

Calories: 250 Cal

Total Fat: 23 g

Saturated Fat: 0 g

Cholesterol: 0 mg

Total Carbs: 9 g

Protein: 14 g

Keto Chaffle Waffle

Preparation time :

Cooking time :

INGREDIENTS :

1 egg

½ cup of shredded mozzarella cheese

1 ½ tablespoon of almond flour

Pinch of baking powder

DIRECTIONS :

Preheat your waffle maker.

In a bowl, whisk the egg and shredded mozzarella cheese together.

Then add the almond powder and baking powder to the bowl and whisk them until the mixture is consistent.

Then pour the mixture onto the centre of the waffle machine.

Close the machine and let the waffles cook until golden brown.

Serve and enjoy.

NUTRITION :

Calories 320

Carbohydrates: 2.9g

Protein: 21.5g

Fat: 24.3g

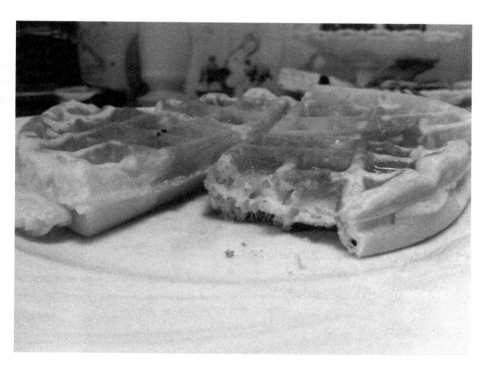

Keto Chaffle Topped with Salted Caramel Syrup

Preparation time : 15 mins

Cooking time : 10 mins

INGREDIENTS :

1 egg

½ cup of mozzarella cheese

¼ cup of cream

2 tablespoon of collagen powder

1 ½ tablespoon of almond flour

1 ½ tablespoon of unsalted butter

Pinch of salt

¾ tablespoon of powdered erythritol

Pinch of baking powder

DIRECTIONS:

Preheat your waffle machine

Whisk together the chaffle ingredients that include the egg, mozzarella cheese, almond flour, and baking powder.

Pour the mixture on the waffle machine. Let it cook until golden brown.

To make the caramel syrup, turn on the flame under a pan to medium heat Melt the unsalted butter on the pan.

Then turn the heat low and add collagen powder and erythritol to the pan and whisk them. Gradually add the cream and remove from heat. Then add the salt and continue to whisk.

Pour the syrup onto the chaffle and enjoy.

NUTRITION :

Calories: 605

Fat: 45g

Protein: 48g

Carbohydrates: 5.1g

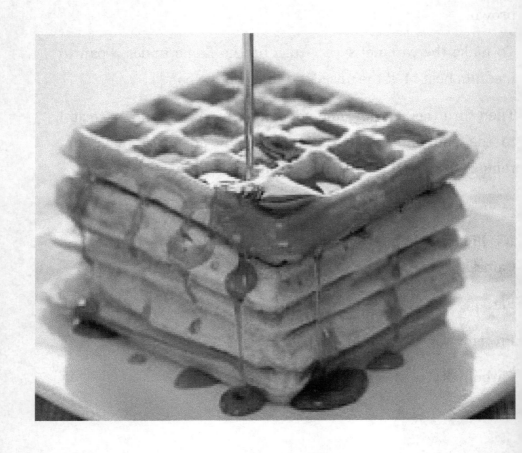

Keto Chaffle Bacon Sandwich

Preparation time : 15 mins

Cooking time : 10 mins

INGREDIENTS :

1 egg

½ cup of shredded mozzarella cheese

2 Tablespoon of coconut flour

2 strips of pork or beef bacon

1 slice of any type of cheese

2 tablespoon of coconut oil

DIRECTIONS:

Preheat your waffle machine.

In a bowl, beat 1 egg, ½ cup of mozzarella cheese, and almond flour. Pour the mixture on the waffle machine. Let it cook until it is golden brown. Then remove it to a plate.

Warm coconut oil in a pan over medium heat. Then place the bacon strips in the pan. Cook until crispy over medium heat. Assemble the bacon and cheese on the chaffle.

NUTRITION :

Calories: 580

Fat: 52g

Carbohydrates: 3g

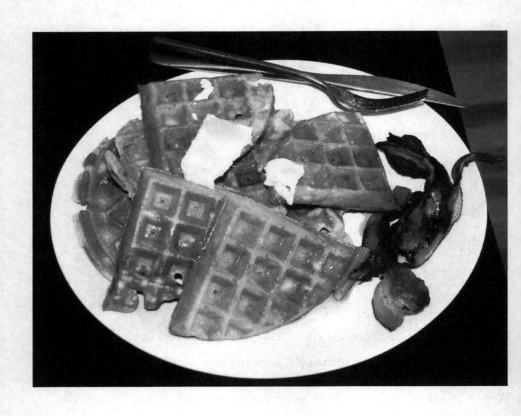

Crispy Zucchini Chaffle

Preparation time : 15 mins

Cooking time : 5 mins

INGREDIENTS :

2 eggs

1 fresh zucchini

1 cup of shredded or grated cheddar cheese

2 pinch of salt

1 tablespoon of onion (chopped)

1 clove of garlic

DIRECTIONS :

Preheat the waffle maker.

Start by dicing onions and mashing the garlic. Then grate the zucchini.

Add 2 eggs and the grated zucchini in a bowl.

Also, add the onions, salt, and garlic for extra flavor. You can also add other herbs to give your zaful a crispy more flavor. Then sprinkle ½ cup of cheese on top of the waffle machine.

Add the mixture from the bowl to the waffle machine. Add the remaining cheese on top of the waffle machine and close the waffle machine. Make sure the waffle cooks for about 3 to 5 minutes until it turns golden brown.

By the layering method, you will achieve the perfect crisp. Take out your zucchini chaffles and serve them hot and fresh.

NUTRITION :

Calories: 170

Fat: 12g

Carbohydrates: 4g

Protein: 11g

Peanut Butter Chaffle

Preparation time : 15 min

Cooking time : 10 min

INGREDIENTS :

1 egg

½ cup of cheddar cheese

2 tablespoon of peanut butter

Few drops of vanilla extract

DIRECTIONS :

Grate some cheddar cheese.

Add one egg, cheddar cheese, 2 tablespoon of peanut butter, and a few drops of vanilla extract and mix thoroughly.

Then sprinkle some shredded cheese as a base on the waffle maker. Pour the mixture on top of the waffle machine.

Sprinkle more cheese on top of the mixture and close the waffle machine. Ensure that the waffle is cooked thoroughly for about a few minutes until they are golden brown. Then remove it and enjoy your deliciously cooked chaffles.

NUTRITION :

Calories: 363kcal

Fat: 29g

Protein: 22g

Carbohydrates: 4g

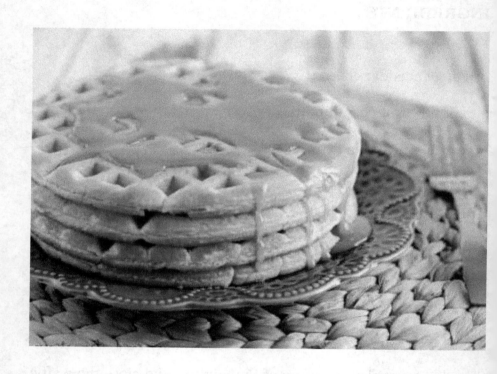

Buffalo hummus beef chaffless

Preparation time : 15 minutes
Cooking time : 32 minutes

Servings : 4
INGREDIENTS :

Two eggs

1 cup + ¼ cup finely grated cheddar cheese, divided

two chopped fresh scallions

Salt

freshly ground black pepper

Two chicken breasts, cooked and diced

¼ cup buffalo sauce

3 tbsp low-carb hummus

Two celery stalks, chopped

¼ cup crumbled blue cheese for topping

DIRECTIONS :

Preheat the waffle iron.

In a medium bowl, mix the eggs, 1 cup of the cheddar cheese, scallions, salt, and black pepper,

Open the iron and add a quarter of the mixture. Close and cook until crispy

Transfer the chaffle to a plate and make three more chaffless in the same manner.

Heat to 400f, the oven and line a parchment paper baking sheet. Set aside.

Cut the chaffless into quarters and arrange on the baking sheet.

In a medium bowl, mix the chicken with the buffalo sauce, hummus, and celery.

Spoon the chicken mixture onto each quarter of chaffless and top with the remaining cheddar cheese.

Position the baking sheet in the oven and bake for 4 minutes, until the cheese melts.

Take out of the oven and top with the blue cheese.

NUTRITION :

Calories: 552Cal

Total Fat: 28.37g

Saturated Fat: 0g

Cholesterol: 0mg

Total Carbs: 6.97 g

Protein: 59.8 g

Cauliflower Turkey Chaffle

Preparation Time : 5 minutes

Cooking Time : 12 minutes

Servings : 2

INGREDIENTS :

One large egg (beaten)

½ cup cauliflower rice

¼ cup diced turkey

½ tsp coconut amino or soy sauce

A pinch of ground black pepper

A pinch of white pepper

¼ tsp curry

¼ tsp oregano

1 tbsp butter (melted)

¾ cup shredded mozzarella cheese

One garlic clove (crushed)

DIRECTIONS :

Preheat the waffle maker and spray.

Combine the cauliflower rice, white pepper, black pepper, curry, and oregano in a mixing dish.

Whisk together the eggs, sugar, crushed garlic, and the coconut amino acid in another mixing cup.

Place the egg mixture into the cheese mixture and thoroughly blend the ingredients.

Stir-in the diced turkey.

Sprinkle 2 tbsp cheese over the waffle maker. Fill the waffle maker with an appropriate amount of the batter. Spread out the mixture to the edges to cover all the holes on the waffle maker. Sprinkle another 2 tbsp cheese over the dough.

Cover the waffle maker and cook for about 4 minutes.

After the cooking cycle, remove the chaffle from the waffle maker.

Repeat steps 6 to 8 until you have cooked all the batter into chaffles.

Serve warm and enjoy.

NUTRITION :
Calories: 168

Total Fat: 11.5g

Saturated Fat: 6.1g

Cholesterol: 127mg

Sodium: 184mg

Total Carbohydrate: 3.8g

Total Sugars: 1.2g

Protein: 12.5g

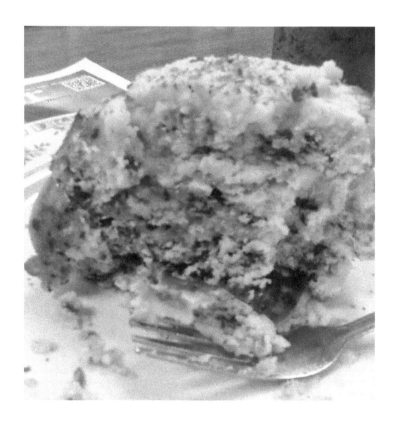

Chaffle with Sausage Gravy

Preparation Time : 10 minutes
Cooking Time : 15 minutes

Servings : 2
INGREDIENTS :

Sausage Gravy:

¼ cup cooked breakfast sausage

1/8 tsp onion powder

1/8 tsp garlic powder

½ tsp pepper or more to taste

3 tbsp chicken broth

2 tsp cream cheese

2 tbsp heavy whipping cream

¼ tsp oregano

Chaffle:

1 tbsp almond flour

1 tbsp finely chopped onion

1/8 tsp salt

¼ tsp baking powder

½ cup mozzarella cheese

1 egg (beaten)

DIRECTIONS :

Preheat the waffle maker and spray.

Combine the almond flour, chopped onion, mozzarella, baking powder, and salt in a mixing bowl. Add the egg and mix until the ingredients are well combined.

Cover and bake for about 4 minutes.

After the baking cycle, remove the chaffle from the waffle maker.

Repeat steps 3 to 5 until you have cooked all the batter into chaffles.

Heat a saucepan over medium or high heat.

Add-in the oregano, garlic powder, onion powder, pepper, cream cheese, and whipped cream to the chicken broth.

Lower the heat after boiling and simmer for about 7 minutes or until the gravy sauce thickens.

Serve the chaffless with the gravy and enjoy it.

NUTRITION :

Total Fat: 16.6g

Saturated Fat 7.3g

Cholesterol 123mg

Sodium 429mg

Total Carbohydrate 3.3g

Dietary Fiber 0.8g

Total Sugars 0.7g

Protein 9.8g

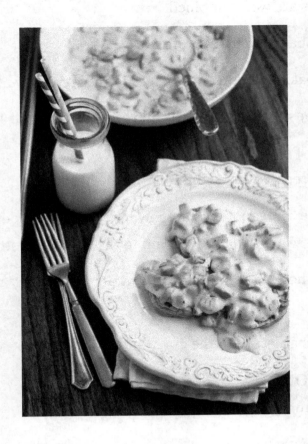

Lobster Chaffle

Preparation Time : 5 minutes

Cooking Time : 8 minutes

Servings : 2

INGREDIENTS :

1 egg (beaten)

½ cup shredded mozzarella cheese

¼ tsp garlic powder

¼ tsp onion powder

1/8 tsp Italian seasoning

Lobster Filling:

½ cup lobster tails (defrosted)

1 tbsp mayonnaise

1 tsp dried basil

1 tsp lemon juice

1 tbsp chopped green onion

DIRECTIONS:

Preheat and spray the waffle maker.

In a mixing bowl, combine the mozzarella, Italian seasoning, garlic, and onion powder. Add the egg and mix until the ingredients are well combined.

Pour an appropriate amount of the batter into the waffle maker and spread out the dough to cover all the holes on the waffle maker.

Cover the waffle maker and cook for about 4 minutes.

After the cooking cycle, remove and transfer the chaff to a wire rack to cool.

Repeat steps 3 to 5 until you have cooked all the batter into chaffless.

For the filling, put the lobster tail in a mixing bowl and add the mayonnaise, basil and lemon juice. Toss until the ingredients are well combined.

Fill the chaffless without the lobster mixture and garnish with chopped green onion.

Serve and enjoy.

NUTRITION :

Total Fat 6.3g

Saturated Fat 1.9g

Cholesterol 141mg

Sodium 303mg

Total Carbohydrate 3g

Dietary Fiber 0.2g

Total Sugars 1g

Protein 11.9g

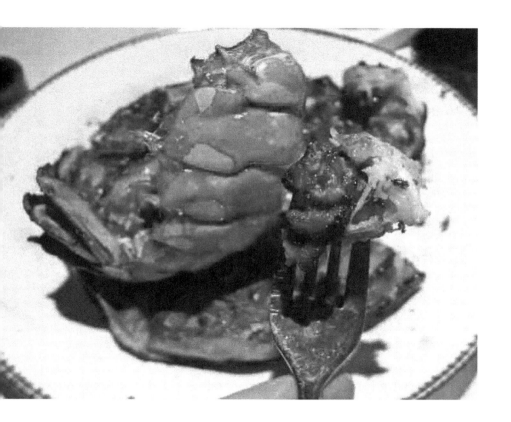

Savory Pork Rind Chaffle

Preparation Time : 5 minutes

Cooking Time : 10 minutes

Servings : 2

INGREDIENTS :

¼ tsp paprika

¼ tsp oregano

¼ tsp garlic powder

½ onion (finely chopped)

½ cup pork rind (crushed)

½ cup mozzarella cheese

1/8 tsp ground black pepper

1 large egg (beaten)

DIRECTIONS :

Preheat and spray the waffle maker.

In a mixing bowl, combine the crushed pork rind, cheese, onion, paprika, garlic powder, and pepper. Add the egg and mix until the ingredients are well combined.

Pour an appropriate amount of the batter into the waffle maker and spread out the dough to cover all the holes on the waffle maker.

Cover the waffle maker and cook for about 5 minutes.

After the cooking cycle, remove the chaffle from the waffle maker.

Repeat steps 3 to 5 until you have cooked all the batter into chaffless.

Serve and top with sour cream as desired.

NUTRITION :

Calories 392

Total Fat 24g

Saturated Fat 9.6g

Cholesterol 177mg

Sodium 1169mg

Total Carbohydrate 3.6g

Total Sugars 1.5g

Protein 41.9g

Smoked salmon

Preparation Time : 10 minutes

Cooking Time : 20 minutes

Servings : 6

INGREDIENTS :

7 ounces of salmon (smoked)

The zest from half of a lemon)

8 ounces of cream cheese

4 tablespoons of dill (fresh)

5 and an additional 1/3 tablespoons of mayo

2 ounces of lettuce

DIRECTIONS :

Cut your salmon into small pieces.

Combine all of your ingredients in a bowl.

Let it sit for 15 minutes.

Place on a lettuce leaf.

NUTRITION :

Calories: 330 Cal

Total Fat: 26 g

Saturated Fat: 0 g

Cholesterol: 0 mg

Total Carbs: 3 g

Protein: 23 g

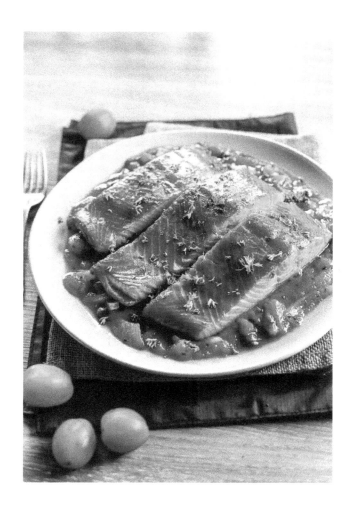

Grilled steak

Preparation Time : 8 minutes

Cooking Time : 17 minutes

Servings : 6

INGREDIENTS:

1 clove of garlic

1tablespoon of oregano (fresh)

½ of a teaspoon of salt

1 tablespoons oil (olive)

¼ of a teaspoon of pepper

¼ of a teaspoon of pepper flakes (red ones)

1 tablespoon lime juice (fresh)

Three diced avocados

Three tablespoons vinegar (used red wine)

2 pounds of flank steak

Pepper

Salt

DIRECTIONS:

Heat a grill to medium-high heat or 400 degrees.

Add all of the ingredients for the sauce to a food processor and blend until smooth.

Add the avocado and the sauce you blended.

Toss lightly, so it gets coated but not hard enough to crush the avocado.

Take a room temperature flank steak and season both sides with pepper and salt.

Remove from your grill and let cool for a few minutes.

Slice the steak and drizzle the top with sauce or serve it on the side.

NUTRITION :

Calories: 444 Cal

Total Fat: 32 g

Saturated Fat: 0 g

Cholesterol: 0 mg

Total Carbs: 7 g

Protein: 34 g

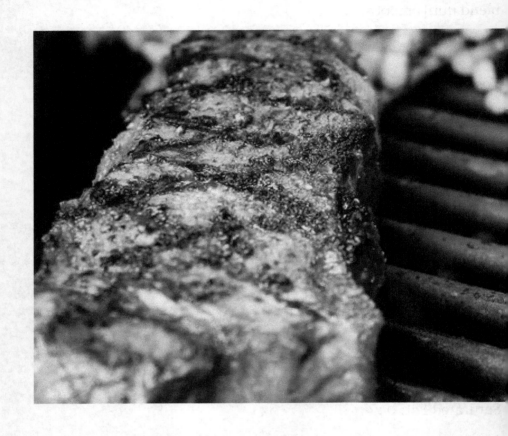

Crab Chaffles

Preparation Time : 10 minutes

Cooking Time : 25 minutes

Servings : 6

INGREDIENTS :

1 lb crab meat

1/3 cup Panko breadcrumbs

One egg

2 tbsp fat greek yoghurt

1 tsp Dijon mustard

2 tbsp parsley and chives, fresh

1 tsp Italian seasoning

One lemon, juiced

Salt, pepper to taste

DIRECTIONS:

Preheat, the waffle maker

Add all ingredients, except the crab meat in a small bowl.

Add the meat. Mix well.

Form the mixture into round patties.

Cook 1 patty for 3 minutes

Remove it and repeat the process with the remaining crab chaffle mixture.

Once ready, remove and enjoy warm.

NUTRITION :

Calories: 99Cal

Total Fat: 8g

Saturated Fat: 0g

Cholesterol: 0mg

Total Carbs: 4g

Protein: 16g

Protein Chaffles

Preparation Time : 3 minutes

Cooking Time : 4 minutes

Servings : 1

INGREDIENTS:

¼ cup almond milk

¼ cup plant-based protein powder

2 tbsp almond butter

1 tbsp psyllium husk

DIRECTIONS:

Preheat the waffle maker.

Combine almond milk, protein powder, psyllium husk, and mix thoroughly until the mixture gets the form of a paste.

Add in butter, combine well and form round balls

Put the ball in the center of the preheated waffle maker.

Cook for 4 minutes.

Remove, top as preferred and enjoy.

NUTRITION :

Calories: 310Cal

Total Fat: 19g

Saturated Fat: 0g

Cholesterol: 0mg

Total Carbs 50g

Protein: 25g

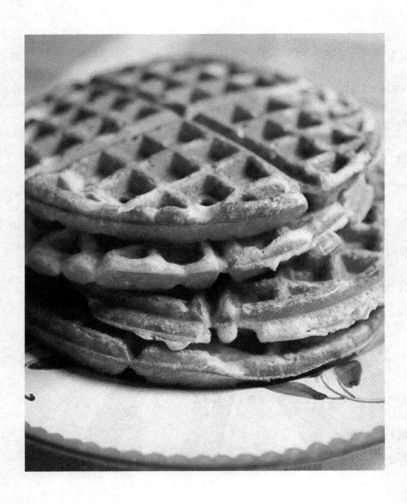

Turnip Hash Brown Chaffles

Preparation time : 10 minutes

Cooking time : 42 minutes

Servings : 6

INGREDIENTS:

1 large turnip, peeled and shredded

½ medium white onion, minced

2 garlic cloves, pressed

1 cup finely grated Gouda cheese

2 eggs, beaten

Salt

freshly ground black pepper

DIRECTIONS:

Pour the turnips in a medium safe microwave bowl, sprinkle with 1 tbsp of water, and steam in the microwave until softened, 1 to 2 minutes.

Remove the bowl and mix in the remaining ingredients except for a quarter cup of the Gouda cheese.

Preheat the waffle iron.

Once heated, open and sprinkle some of the reserved cheese in the iron and top with 3 tablespoons of the mixture. Close the waffle iron and cook until crispy, 5 minutes.

Open the lid, flip the chaffle and cook further for 2 more minutes.

Remove the chaffle onto a plate and set aside.

Make five more chaffles with the remaining batter in the same proportion.

Allow cooling and serve afterward.

NUTRITION :

Calories: 99 Cal

Total Fat: 8 g

Saturated Fat: 0 g

Cholesterol: 0 mg

Total Carbs: 4 g

Everything Bagel Chaffles

Preparation time : 10 minutes
Cooking time : 28 minutes

Servings : 4

INGREDIENTS:

1 egg, beaten

½ cup finely grated Parmesan cheese

1 tsp Everything Bagel seasoning

DIRECTIONS:

Preheat the waffle iron.

Combine all the ingredients in a bowl.

Open the iron, pour in a quarter of the mixture, close, and cook until crispy, 6 to 7 minutes.

Remove the chaffle onto a plate and set aside.

Make three more chaffles, allow cooling, and enjoy after.

NUTRITION :

Calories: 99 Cal

Total Fat: 8 g

Saturated Fat: 0 g

Cholesterol: 0 mg

Total Carbs: 4 g

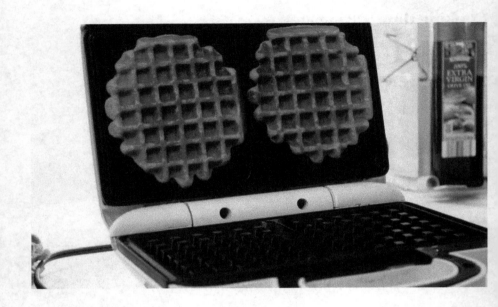

Blueberry Shortcake Chaffles

Preparation time : 10 minutes

Cooking time : 14 minutes

Servings : 2

INGREDIENTS :

1 egg, beaten

1 tbsp cream cheese, softened

¼ cup finely grated mozzarella cheese

1/4 tsp baking powder

4 fresh blueberries

1 tsp blueberry extract

DIRECTIONS:

Preheat the waffle iron.

Combine all the ingredients in a bowl.

Open the iron, pour in half of the batter, close, and cook until crispy, 6 to 7 minutes.

Remove the chaffle onto a plate and set aside.

Make the other chaffle with the remaining batter.

Allow cooling and enjoy after.

NUTRITION :

Calories: 99 Cal

Total Fat: 8 g

Saturated Fat: 0 g

Cholesterol: 0 mg

Total Carbs: 4 g

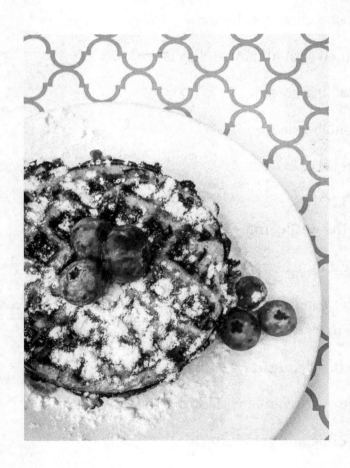

Raspberry-Pecan Chaffles

Preparation time : 10 minutes

Cooking time : 14 minutes

Servings : 2

INGREDIENTS :

1 egg, beaten

½ cup finely grated mozzarella cheese

1 tbsp cream cheese, softened

1 tbsp sugar-free maple syrup

¼ tsp raspberry extract

¼ tsp vanilla extract

2 tbsp sugar-free caramel sauce for topping

3 tbsp chopped pecans for topping

DIRECTIONS:

Preheat the waffle iron.

Combine all ingredients in a small bowl.

Open the iron, pour in half of the batter, close, and cook until crispy, 6 to 7 minutes.

Remove the chaffle onto a plate and set aside.

Make another chaffle with the remaining batter.

To serve: drizzle the caramel sauce on the chaffles and top with the pecans.

NUTRITION :

Calories: 99 Cal

Total Fat: 8 g

Saturated Fat: 0 g

Cholesterol: 0 mg

Total Carbs: 3 g

Scrambled Egg Stuffed Chaffles

Preparation time : 15 minutes

Cooking time : 28 minutes

Servings : 4

INGREDIENTS :

For the chaffles:

1 cup finely grated cheddar cheese

2 eggs, beaten

For the egg stuffing:

1 tbsp olive oil

4 large eggs

1 small green bell pepper, chopped

1 small red bell pepper

Salt

freshly ground black pepper

2 tbsp grated Parmesan cheese

DIRECTIONS:

For the chaffles:

Preheat the waffle iron.

In a medium bowl, mix the cheddar cheese and egg.

Open the iron, pour in a quarter of the mixture, close, and cook until crispy, 6 to 7 minutes.

Plate and make three more chaffles using the remaining mixture.

For the egg stuffing:

Meanwhile, heat the olive oil in a medium skillet over medium heat on a stovetop.

Beat the eggs with the bell peppers, salt, black pepper, and Parmesan cheese in a medium dish.

Pour the mixture into the skillet and scramble until set to your likeness, 2 minutes.

Between two chaffles, spoon half of the scrambled eggs and repeat with the second set of chaffles.

Serve afterward.

NUTRITION :
Calories: 99 Cal

Total Fat: 8 g

Saturated Fat: 0 g

Cholesterol: 0 mg

Total Carbs: 4 g

Mixed Berry-Vanilla Chaffles

Preparation time : 10 minutes

Cooking time : 28 minutes

Servings : 4

INGREDIENTS :

1 egg, beaten

½ cup finely grated mozzarella cheese

1 tbsp cream cheese, softened

1 tbsp sugar-free maple syrup

2 strawberries, sliced

2 raspberries, slices

¼ tsp blackberry extract

¼ tsp vanilla extract

½ cup plain yogurt for serving

DIRECTIONS:

Preheat the waffle iron.

Combine all the ingredients in a medium container except the yogurt.

Open the iron, lightly grease with cooking spray and pour in a quarter of the mixture.

Close the iron and cook until golden brown and crispy, 7 minutes.

Remove the chaffle onto a plate and set aside.

Make three more chaffles with the remaining mixture.

To serve: top with the yogurt and enjoy.

NUTRITION :

Calories: 99 Cal

Total Fat: 8 g

Saturated Fat: 0 g

Cholesterol: 0 mg

Total Carbs: 4 g

Ham and Cheddar Chaffles

Preparation time : 15 minutes

Cooking time : 28 minutes

Servings : 4

INGREDIENTS:

1 cup finely shredded parsnips, steamed

8 oz ham, diced

2 eggs, beaten

1 ½ cups finely grated cheddar cheese

½ tsp garlic powder

2 tbsp chopped fresh parsley leaves

¼ tsp smoked paprika

½ tsp dried thyme

Salt

freshly ground black pepper

DIRECTIONS:

Preheat the waffle iron.

Mix all ingredients in a medium container.

Open the iron, lightly grease with cooking spray and pour in a quarter of the mixture.

Close the iron and cook until crispy, 7 minutes.

Remove the chaffle onto a plate and set aside.

Make three more chaffles using the remaining mixture.

Serve afterward.

NUTRITION :

Calories: 99Cal

Total Fat: 8g

Saturated Fat: 0g

Cholesterol: 0mg

Total Carbs: 4g

Savory Gruyere and Chives Chaffles

Preparation time : 15 minutes

Cooking time : 14 minutes

Servings : 2

INGREDIENTS:

2 eggs, beaten

1 cup finely grated Gruyere cheese

2 tbsp finely grated cheddar cheese

1/8 tsp freshly ground black pepper

3 tbsp minced fresh chives + more for garnishing

2 sunshine fried eggs for topping

DIRECTIONS:

Preheat the waffle iron.

In a medium bowl, mix the eggs, cheeses, black pepper, and chives.

Open the iron and pour in half of the mixture.

Close the iron and cook until brown and crispy, 7 minutes.

Remove the chaffle onto a plate and set aside.

Make another chaffle using the remaining mixture.

Top each chaffle with one fried egg each, garnish with the chives and serve.

NUTRITION :

Calories: 99Cal

Total Fat: 8g

Saturated Fat: 0g

Cholesterol: 0mg

Total Carbs: 4g

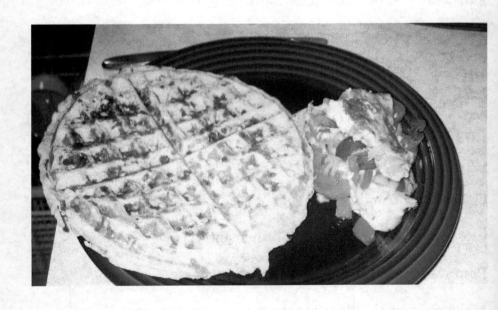

CPSIA information can be obtained
at www.ICGtesting.com
Printed in the USA
BVHW092217260621
610449BV00003B/646